YOUR KNOWLEDGE HAS VALUE

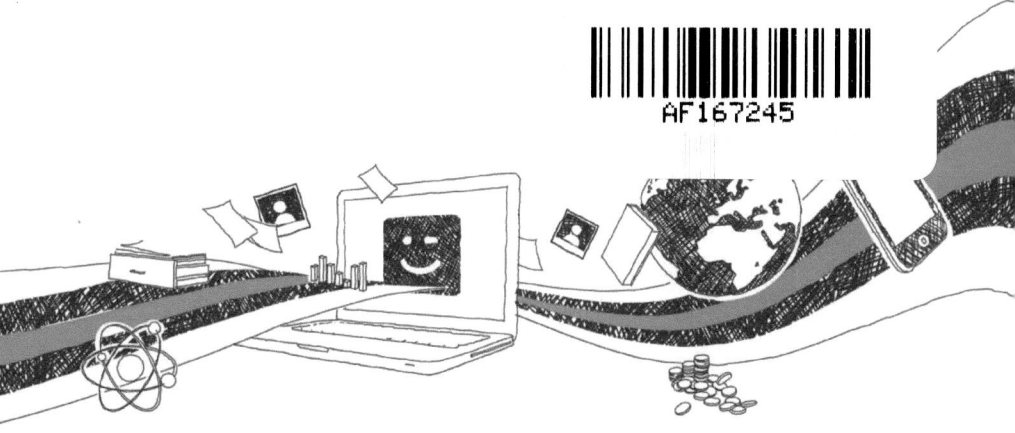
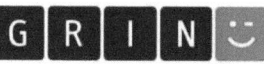

Substance Use in Nigeria

Akinmayowa Adedoyin Shobo

GRIN ☺

Bibliographic information published by the German National Library:

The German National Library lists this publication in the National Bibliography; detailed bibliographic data are available on the Internet at http://dnb.dnb.de.

ISBN: 9783346605757
This book is also available as an ebook.

Print and binding: Books on Demand GmbH, Norderstedt, Germany
Printed on acid-free paper from responsible sources.

The present work has been carefully prepared. Nevertheless, authors and publishers do not incur liability for the correctness of information, notes, links and advice as well as any printing errors.

GRIN web shop: https://www.grin.com/document/1175570

Substance Use and Drug Addiction in Nigeria: An Overview

Abstract

The work is focused on the subject of substance use and drug addiction in Nigeria. The sub-sections explored the existing landscape of substance use/drug abuse domestically and globally while discussing the illicit use of psychoactive substances and their global health implications. Lastly, management of drug addiction was treated.

In Nigeria for instance, there have been growing concerns from various stakeholders from parents of drugs addicts to government regulatory agencies on the burden of drug abuse. The scourge of substance abuse is not limited to the individual; till date its far-reaching implications continues to fuel organized crime, illicit financial flows, corruption, and terrorism/insurgency among others.

There is therefore, need for more proactive steps to eliminate substance use problems across various demographics across the country. Interventions should also be considered amid social, cultural and economic variables that persistently stimulate the behaviour.

Introduction

Nigeria, located in West Africa (depicted below in figure 1) is known for its diversity, having hundreds of ethnicities spread within its borders (Flinders University, 2020). As one visits the local market in rural and urban centres in Nigeria, it is not uncommon to be received by an attractive resplendent display of medicinal substances on stalls, tray or in baskets hawked by mobile sellers. These medicines are mostly in common forms such as plant-based products (powder, suspension, infusion, decoction) while others are largely synthesized pharmaceutical products (such as tablets, capsules, ointment, intravenous (IV) infusions) to mention a few. Interestingly, this open display of medicinal formulations is not limited to the informal settings such as the popular local markets; medicinal agents can be sourced from formal institutions such as pharmacy stores of healthcare institutions and proprietary patent medicine vendors. An important point to note here, is in how medicinal substances (often erroneously called *drugs*) within the health industry are being regulated within a particular territory – in this case, Nigeria. Meanwhile, it is important to highlight that in this work, the term 'substance' is referred to as 'drug' and 'psychoactive drugs'.

The figure has been removed for copyright reasons

Figure 1: map of Nigeria

As alluded earlier, drugs are often exploited for their therapeutic benefits. Such benefits ranging from disease treatment to general maintenance of good health and well-being. In the same manner, there are certain category of drugs that are exploited for their potential to alter the mental and psychological states of individuals.

3

Often they are harnessed for management of psychological disorders such as depressive disorders, sleep disorders, nociception. Yet some of these drugs are used for recreational purposes. In many societies, there has been intense debate of benefits and harm of these 'psychoactive' drugs. This is owing to the link between the consumption of substances and detrimental costs to individuals and their society at last. This is aptly termed under the subject matter of drug abuse or substance use.

By definition, as reported in Jatau et al. (2021), Drug abuse is "... the use of a drug that is not generally accepted on medical ground, i.e. continuous or occasional use of drugs that would cause overt behavioral change by the individual either of his own choice or under a feeling of compulsion, to achieve his wellbeing or what he conceives as of his own wellbeing" (Benjamin & Chidi, 2014).

From available literature, the dangers of substance abuse have been studied for its impact in child development particularly between the phases of adolescence and young adulthood. It has been described as a "chronic debilitating disease with significant morbidity and mortality" which affects caregivers and the community at large (Abdullabi & Sarmest, 2019). Drug abuse has been known be non-discriminatory while consumption is associated with increased tendency for crime among young people and an array of health problems (Abdullabi & Sarmest, 2019). As a matter of fact, as indicated by the Diagnostic and Statistical Manual of Mental Disorders (DSM-V) (fifth edition) (cited in Abdullabi & Sarmest, 2019) researchers have been able to characterize a cluster of cognitive, behavioural and physiological symptoms that often accompany many drug abuse-related problems.

In Nigeria for instance, there have been growing concern from various stakeholders from parents of drugs addicts to government regulatory agencies on the burden of drug abuse (Ohuabunwa, 2019). The war against substance use in Nigeria backed by federal laws commenced as far back as 1935. "Some of the most important laws against the cultivation, trafficking, and abuse of illicit drugs in Nigeria are as follows: (a) The Dangerous Drugs Ordinance of 1935 enacted by the British Colonial administration. (b) The Indian Hemp Decree No. 19 of 1966. (c) The Indian Hemp (Amendment) Decree No. 34 of 1979. (d) The Indian Hemp (Amendment) Decree, and the Special Tribunal (Miscellaneous Offences) Decree No. 20 of 1984. (e) The Special Tribunal (Miscellaneous Offences) (Amendment) Decree of 1986 and the National Drug Law Enforcement Agency Decree No. 48 of 1989 (as amended by Decree No.33 of 1990, Decree No 15 of 1992 and Decree No. 62 of 1999). These laws were harmonized as an Act of the parliament, CAP N30 Laws of the Federation of Nigeria (LFN) 2004. This Act established the NDLEA." (NDLEA, 2020; Jatau et al., 2021).

From an epidemiological standpoint, drug abuse is fast attaining epidemic status. For instance; the Global Burden of disease Study estimated that, in 2017, there were 585,000 deaths owing to drug use, globally (UNODC, 2019). Further, a report by the United Nations Office on Drugs and Crime (UNODC) has projected that 35 million individuals will be experiencing drug use disorders (UNODC, 2019). The cost of problems arising from substance use (in the form of usage, abuse, and trafficking) has been profiled under four main dimensions namely "organized crime, illicit financial flows, corruption, and terrorism/insurgency" (UNODC, 2017).

In Nigeria, the burden of drug abuse is also dire. According to a 2018 UNODC report on "Drug use in Nigeria" (a nationwide drug use survey), it was estimated that "... 1 in 7 individuals (aged 15–64 years) had been involved in substance use in the past year (UNODC, 2018). Further, 1 in 5 persons who had used drug in the past year is suffering from drug-associated disorders (UNODC, 2018).

Consequently, there's an urgent need for research on practical interventions at domestic and global levels to mitigate the scourge of drug abuse and its associated implications on health, governance, and security matters.

Review of empirical studies

Although there have been several scholarly works on substance use; by conducting a systemic review, Jatau and co-researchers highlighted elements of the most current status about the subject in Nigeria. The study aimed at summarizing the findings from epidemiological studies on drug abuse and provision of drug laws in Nigeria (Jatau et al., 2021). The cluster of epidemiological studies covered a wide range of demography including secondary school students (Famuyiwa et al., 2011; Erah and Omatseye, 2017; Abdulkarim et al., 2005; Lawoyin et al., 2005), drug abusers (Adamson et al., 2010; Dankani, 2012), undergraduate students (Essien, 2010; Makanjuola et al., 2007), members of several communities (Gobir et al., 2017; Namadi, 2016; UNODC, 2018), commercial vehicle drivers (Makanjuola et al., 2007; Yunusa et al., 2017).

In terms of prevalence of drug abuse in Nigeria; findings from 23 epidemiological studies revealed a prevalence of "... revealed between 20 and 40% among the secondary school students; 20.9% among youths in the community and 81.1% among commercial bus drivers."

Concerning the epidemiology of the commonly abused drugs in Nigeria; the study found the following drugs were most frequently used within the population: cannabis, codeine, amphetamine/ dexamphetamine, heroin, cocaine, diazepam, and cough syrup, Reactivan (fencamfamine), Mandrax, Madrax (Methadone and diphenhydramine), Proplus (caffeine 50 mg) and tramadol.

Additionally, cannabis was the most abused drug reported across the different study populations. The prevalence of cannabis abuse among members of the general public was 10.8% and 22.7% among adolescents of 25 years and younger. The frequency of abuse among secondary school students was as high as 34% in some cases. The frequency of cocaine abuse ranges from 1.6 to 4.8% among secondary school students, 0.6–10% among undergraduate students and 0.1–0.6% among members of the general public.

Codeine was the third most frequently reported drug of abuse from the included studies. The prevalence of abuse was 22.7% among adolescent; 8.2% among undergraduate students and 28% among secondary school students.

Further, the study also investigated sources of the drugs available to abusers in Nigeria. There include: pharmacies/patent medicine shops (23–33%), open markets (17%), drug hawkers, hawkers of traditional herbal preparations, fellow drug abusers (8%), underground agents (57%), family members (1.6–33%), friends (up to 61%), teachers (3%), physician (8.3%), other health practitioners (3.0%).

From the population, some of the reasons responsible for abuse of drugs include: increase physical performance, pleasure, desire to relax/sleep, experiment/curiosity, maintain wakefulness, reduce stress, as anti-anxiety, unemployment, frustration, and easy access. In agreement with the study result, Jatau and the other authors noted that "... the high poverty rate of about 50% of people living in extreme poverty in Nigeria (The World Bank, 2020), and the rising rate of unemployment (23.1%) (National Bureau of Statistics, 2019) may worsen the socioeconomic conditions of Nigerians; further contributing to the predisposition to substance use. Hence; people consume these drugs for example; to combat stress levels.

Other associated variables that increase the risk of drug abuse was also revealed including: gender (male), poor economic status, parental deprivation (dysfunctional family), education level, and peer-group influence. For instance; age was a strong predictor, as the study reported that "...younger population (less than 35 years) was the most affected group by substance use among other groups" (ibid).

Psychoactive Substances: The Pharmacology

As defined by the World Health Organisation (WHO); psychoactive substances (or drugs), are "substances that have the potential to elicit changes in an individual's consciousness, affect or thinking processes" (WHO, 2004). In many countries, the use of psychoactive substances is regulated by socio-legal structures; hence, their categorisation. As indicated below, there are several psychoactive substances that have received huge patronage including caffeine, nicotine, alcoholic beverages. There are also many widely consumed agents that have commonly abused (or misused) (in spite of the prohibited status) such as cannabis, opiates, hallucinogens among others.

First, as pharmacotherapy. Here, there are evidences that argue in favour of the therapeutic benefits of these substances in the treatment of neurological and psychological disorders in many global indigenous systems of medicine. Under orthodox system of medicine, these use of psychoactive agents are constrained to a physician's orders, via a "prescription system.". For example; the use of methylphenidate and ADHD.

The second category is in terms of its illicit, non-medical use. Under at least three international conventions, countries agree to "prohibit trade in and non-medical use of opiates, cannabis, hallucinogens, cocaine and many other stimulants, and many hypnotics and sedatives." The conventions include the *single Convention on Narcotic Drugs, 1961; Convention on Psychotropic Substances, 1971; United Nations Convention against Illicit Traffic in Narcotic Drugs and Psychotropic Substances, 1988* (UNODC, 2002). Interestingly, there is literature that posit that in spite of the prohibitions and other control measures, these substances may continue to receive wide patronage for non-medical purposes owing to, perhaps the *attractive frisson* phenomenon among users.

Lastly, there is a third category of consumption that has a legal status. For instance; the use of "an alcoholic beverage can be a source of nutrition, of heating or cooling the body, or of thirst-quenching; or for religious purposes". Here, the fundamental purpose is not for the psychoactive effect.

In a bid to understand the broader implications of psychoactive substances use and its negative extreme, its misuse and abuse; it is relevant to highlight the fundamental physiological processes underlying the action of the drugs at the neurological level.

In a systemic review reported in Jatau et al (2021), it was stressed from various epidemiological studies on drug abuse in Nigeria that the most commonly abused psychoactive substance (for illicit use) include *cannabis* (highest rank i.e. 10.8% among members of the general public and 22.7% among adolescents), *codeine, cocaine, heroin, amphetamine, diazepam, tramadol* among others (Namadi, 2016Yunusa et al., 2017; UNODC, 2018). Hence, the psychopharmacology of cannabis is highlighted below.

Cannabis/cannabinoids:

The figure has been removed for copyright reasons

Figure 2: Cannabis sativa (source: www.googleimages.com)

Asides its potential for abuse, in many regions of the world, cannabis has been exploited for its medical uses including as an adjunct drug in the treatment of nausea among cancer patients. Of the cannabinoids contained in *Cannabis sativa* (depicted above in figure 2), δ-9-tetrahydrocannabinol (THC) is the major chemical with psychoactive effects and is metabolized to another active compound, 11-OH-δ-9-THC. "Cannabinoids are generally inhaled by smoking, but may also be ingested. Peak intoxication through smoking is reached within 15–30 minutes and the effects last for 2–6 hours. Cannabinoids remain in the body for long periods and accumulate after repeated use."

Some of the behavioural effect of cannabis include: euphoria, altered perception of time (slow), relaxation, sharpened sensory awareness, analgesia, increased appetite among others (O´Brien, 2001; WHO, 2004).

Mechanism of action: Using receptor pharmacology, cannabinoid receptors and their endogenous ligands together constitute what is now referred to as the 'endocannabinoid system'. "Cannabinoid compounds induce their pharmacological effects by activating two different receptors that have been identified and cloned: the CB-1 cannabinoid receptor, which is highly expressed in the central nervous system (Devane et al., 1988; Matsuda et al., 1990; WHO, 2004), and the CB-2 cannabinoid receptor, which is localized in the peripheral tissues mainly at the level of the immune system (Munro, Thomas & Abu-Shaar, 1993; WHO, 2004)."

"The CB1 receptors located at nerve terminals (Pertwee, 1997; Ong & Mackie, 1999; Pertwee, 2001) suppress the neuronal release of transmitters that include acetylcholine, noradrenaline, dopamine, 5-hydroxy-tryptamine, GABA, glutamate and aspartate (Pertwee, 2001). CB2 receptors found in immune cells, with particularly high levels in B-cells and natural killer cells (Galiegue et al., 1995), are immunomodulatory (Molina-Holgado, Lledo & Guaza, 1997)."

As characteristic of many psychoactive substances; there is the risk of drug tolerance upon sustained use due to its action at the CB1 cannabinoid receptor; and the eventual dependence (physical and psychological) (Johns, 2001, WHO, 2004). Additional, the use of cannabis has been linked to "exacerbation of schizophrenic symptoms, long-lasting cognitive impairment (owing to withdrawal reaction or direct neurotoxicity of cannabinoids, tar, carboxyhaemoglobin or benzopyrene)." A review of the preclinical literature suggests that both age during exposure and duration of exposure may be critical determinants of neurotoxicity (Scallet, 1991).

Drug addiction and their implications

There's been extensive scholarly work that establish a multiplicity of effects owing to drug abuse; this is asides the fact that the knowledge of the pathophysiology of substance dependence keeps advancing. The World Drug Report documented that "...1/10 of individuals on illicit substances suffer from some form of dependence." (2012). In another way, these drugs have been found to elicit classic patterns of the addiction pathway including habituation and altered consciousness (Abdullahi and Sarmast, 2019).

Substance addiction (or dependence) has been described as a "compulsive pattern of consumption characterized by loss of control and sustained use of the substance in spite of the biologically significant abuse-related problems and the emergence of a state of physiological need such that a physiological signs and symptoms known as withdrawal symptoms occur when access to the substance is inhibited" (WHO, 2004; UNODC, 2015).

Most addictions are characterized by the following attributes: *experimentation* (or the use of the substance without behavior modification); *regular pattern of use*; *abuse* (marked by craving, pre-occupation with the drugs, depressive symptoms); *physical and/or psychological dependence* (marked by compulsive use of the drug despite severe negative consequences with occurrence of withdrawal symptoms) (Barangam et al., 2007; Barrett et al., 2008).

Conversely, researchers have linked several biological and non-biological factors that could contribute to drug addiction. There include: "genetic predisposition; psychological factors (such as stress, personality traits like high impulsivity, depression, anxiety, eating disorder, personality and other psychiatric disorder); age at first exposure; environmental factors (like availability of drugs, social status, peer pressure, drug awareness like advertisement, sexual abuse or addiction in the family) (O'Brien et al., 1998; Kreek et al., 2005; Abdullabi and Sarmast, 2019)."

As indicated earlier, substance dependence has been linked to various adverse effects. The mechanism of toxicity leading to psychotropic and non-psychotropic effect is depicted in the figure 3 below.

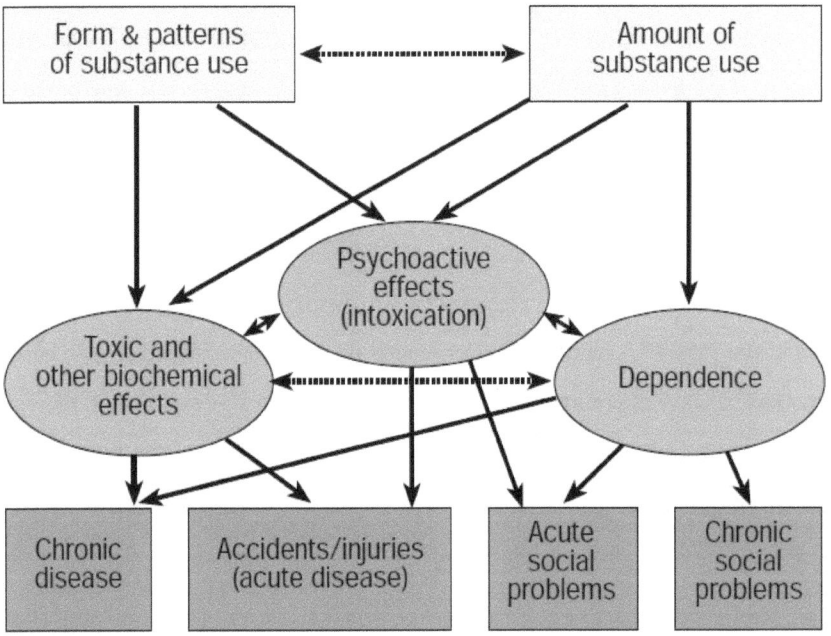

Figure 3: Mechanisms of Toxicity of Substance Use (Source: WHO, 2004)

Additionally, a systematic review of more than 23 epidemiological studies conducted by Jatau and other researchers on drug abuse in Nigeria found several mental health-related features of psychoactive drug intoxication including toxic psychosis, anxiety state, schizophrenia, delusion (Jatau et al., 2021).

Management of Drug Addiction/Substance Use

It is often said that the best form of solution is prevention. Experts have highlighted the importance of delineating the etiology of the global burden of abuse as a means of adopting prevention approaches including community education programmes (and other interventions) drawn out to bring awareness to the hazards of drug abuse (or misuse) suited for various segment of the Nigerian population notably children of drug addicts. A number of programmes have been recommended such as "[childhood education, parenting skill, behavioural couple therapy, contingency management therapy, cognitive behavior and skill training therapy, family-based therapy]" (Botvin et al., 2001; Carroll & Onkan, 2005; Farell and Schein, 2011). Summarily, there's need for robust health promotion initiatives targeted at (a) enhancing positive health behaviours among this various segments and (b) discouraging negative health behaviours focused on personality, behaviours and environment through community organization, educational interventions and health behavior campaigns (Pentz et al., 2009; Abdullahi and Sarmask, 2019).

Due to the interactive nature of the factors (social, psychological, physiological) influencing substances abuse; other preventative measure may include focus on "... provision of recreational facilities for youths in rural and urban areas, moral rearmament that de-emphasize materialism, improved employment opportunities and effective control of drug availability as well as drug education as part of school curriculum" (Abdullahi and Sarmask, 2019).

From a holistic perspective, patients' care should involve a combinatorial approach using the following modalities: "pharmacotherapy, outpatient counselling-based care and therapeutic communities" (Sindelar & Fiedllin, 2001; Abdullahi and Sarmask, 2019).

- In terms of pharmacotherapy; endogenous receptor blockers (or antagonists) and less potent drug substitutes e.g. methadone maintenance, a synthetic narcotic for heroin and other opiates abuse or Naltrexone, a fast-acting opiate antagonists.
- The counselling programme for treating drug addicts could include psychotherapy, peer counselling.
- Therapeutic community on the other hand, is a programme that emphasizes socialization, life style modifications and behavioural change (Sindelar & Fiedllin, 2001).

Conclusion

The shortfall in addressing the challenges of substance use (or drug abuse) bears a huge toll on individuals, their families and the larger society. As indicated earlier, there's been efforts made locally and globally in the form of development and implementation of policies on the control of illicit substances, and a suite of health promotion programmes. There is however, need for more proactive steps to eliminate substance use problems across various demographics particularly, amid social, cultural and economic variables that persistently stimulate the behaviour.

In Nigeria, studies have mentioned that the widespread use of illicit substances is not unconnected to the ease of access, increased trafficking, lack of policy implementation on drug control and demography-sensitive educational interventions among others. One approach that has been suggested in a bid to reduce the current prevalence of drug abuse is build strong institutions that can cut-off the supply chain of illicit drug trade to the vulnerable segments of the populations.

References

Abdallah, MM (2019). Text of the pre-event press briefing to flag-off the commemoration of 2019 international day against drug abuse and illicit drug trafficking. Available at: https://www.vanguardngr.com/2019/06/drug-abusendleatakes-campaign-to-streets-markets-schools-chairman/ (Accessed: 03/01/2022).

Abdulkarim, AA, Mokuolu, OA, and Adeniyi, A (2005). Drug use among adolescents in Ilorin, Nigeria. Trop Doct. 35 (4), 225–228. doi:10.1258/004947505774938620.

Abdullahi A.M., Sarmast S.T. (2019). Substance Abuse: A Literature Review of the Implications and Solutions. International Journal of Scientific & Engineering Research 10 (10): 1233-1238. ISSN 2229-5518.

Abiodun, O (1991). Drug abuse and its clinical implications with special reference to Nigeria. Cent Afr J Med. 37 (1), 24–30.

Adamson, TA, Onifade, PO, and Ogunwale, A (2010). Trends in sociodemographic and drug abuse variables in patients with alcohol and drug use disorders in a Nigerian treatment facility. W Afr J Med. 29 (1), 12–18. doi:10.4314/wajm.v29i1.55947.

Adelekan, ML, Ogunlesi, AO, and Akindele, MO (1992). Nigerian secondary school teachers: a pilot survey of views and knowledge about drug abuse. East Afr Med J. 69 (3), 140–145.

Akpala, C, and Bolaji, I (1991). Drug abuse among secondary school students in Sokoto, Nigeria. Psychopathol Afr. 23, 197–204.

Benjamin A., Chidi N. (2014). Drug abuse, addiction and dependence, pharmacology and therapeutics, sivakumar joghi thatha gowder, IntechOpen. Available from: https://www.intechopen.com/books/pharmacology-andtherapeutics/

Bramer, WM, Rethlefsen, ML, Kleijnen, J, and Franco, OH (2017). Optimal database combinations for literature searches in systematic reviews: a prospective exploratory study. Syst Rev. 6 (1), 245. doi:10.1186/s13643-017-0644-y.

Dankani, I (2012). Abuse of cough syrups: a new trend in drug abuse in northwestern Nigerian states of Kano, Sokoto, Katsina, Zamfara and Kebbi. Int J Phys Soc Sci. 2 (8), 199–213.

Erah, F, and Omatseye, A (2017). Drug and alcohol abuse among secondary school students in a rural community in south-south Nigeria. Ann Med and Surg Pract. 2 (2), 85–91.

Essien, CF (2010). Drug use and abuse among students in tertiary institutions-the case of federal university of technology, Minna. JORIND. 8 (1), 35–42.

Famuyiwa, O, Aina, OF, and Bankole-Oki, OM (2011). Epidemiology of psychoactive drug use amongst adolescents in metropolitan Lagos, Nigeria. Eur Child Adolesc Psychiatr. 20 (7), 351–359. doi:10.1007/s00787-011-0180-6

Flinders University (2020). The AACODS checklist. Available at: https://dspace.flinders.edu.au/xmlui/bitstream/handle/2328/3326/AACODS_ Checklist.pdf?sequence_4 (Accessed: 03/01/2022).

Gobir, A, Sambo, M, Bashir, S, Olorukoba, A, Ezeh, O, Bello, M, et al. (2017). Prevalence and determinants of drug abuse among youths in A rural community in north western Nigeria. Trop J Health Sci. 24 (4), 5–8.

Jatau AI, Sha'aban A, Gulma KA, Shitu Z, Khalid GM, Isa A, Wada AS and Mustapha M (2021). The Burden of Drug Abuse in Nigeria: A Scoping Review of Epidemiological Studies and Drug Laws. Public Health Rev. 42:1603960. doi: 10.3389/phrs.2021.1603960.

Makanjuola, AB, Daramola, TO, and Obembe, AO (2007). Psychoactive substance use among medical students in a Nigerian university. World Psychiatr. 6 (2), 112–114.

Namadi, MM (2016). Drug abuse among adolescents in Kano metropolis, Nigeria. IJASS. 2 (1), 195–206. doi:10.11648/j.ajns.20170602.16.

National Bureau of Statistics (2019). Unemployment rate 2019. Available at: https://www.nigerianstat.gov.ng/ (Accessed: 03/01/2022).

National Drug Laws Enforcement Agency (2020). Available at: https://nigeriatradeportal.org/media/NDLEA%20Act.pdf (Accessed Accessed: 03/01/2022).

Pela, OA., and Ebie, JC (1982). Drug abuse in Nigeria: a review of epidemiological studies. Bull Narc. 34 (3-4), 91–99.

The World Bank (2020). Poverty and equity data portal—Nigeria. Available at: http://povertydata.worldbank.org/poverty/country/NGA (Accessed: 03/01/2022).

United Nations Office on Drugs and Crime (2017). The drug problem and organized crime, illicit financial flows, corruption and terrorism. Vienna, Austria: United Nations.

United Nations Office on Drugs and Crime (2018). Drug use in Nigeria. Available at: https://www.unodc.org/documents/data-and-analysis/statistics/Drugs/Drug_Use_Survey_Nigeria_2019_BOOK.pdf (Accessed 03 18, 2020).

United Nations Office on Drugs and Crime (UNODC) (2019). World drug report 2019. Available at: https://wdr.unodc.org/wdr2019/en/exsum.html (Accessed: 03/01/2022).

Yunusa U, Bello, UL, Idris M, Haddad MM, and Adamu D (2017).Determinants of substance abuse among commercial bus drivers in Kano Metropolis, Kano State, Nigeria. Ajns. 6 (2), 125–130. doi:10.11648/j.ajns.20170602.16

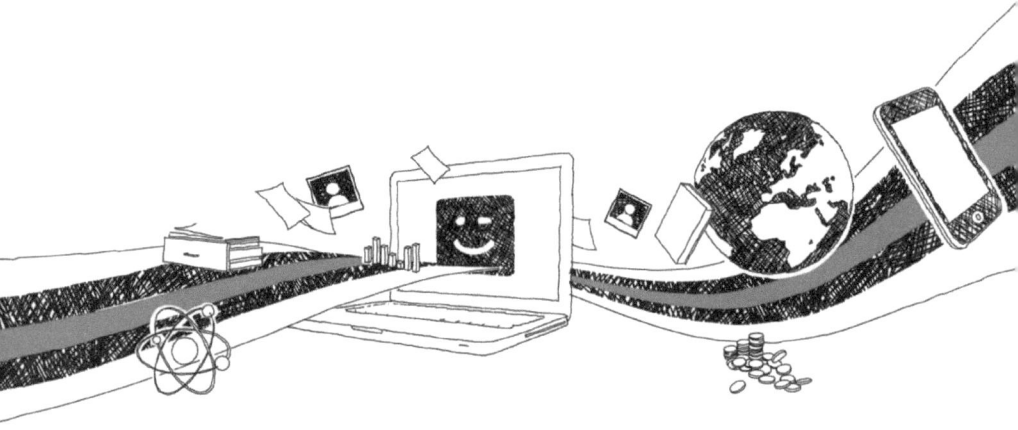